The Healthy Renal Diet Cookbook

Complete, Healthy and Tasty Recipes for Newly Diagnosed Made by Low Sodium, Potassium, and Phosphorus. Start Now to Eat and Feel Healthier

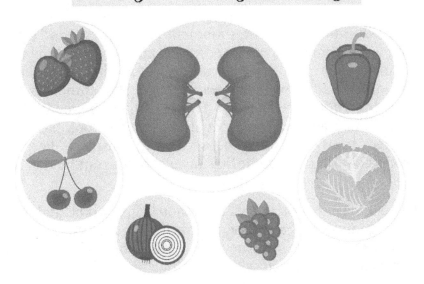

Healthy food for your kidneys

Dylan Ross

Table of Content

Lunch Recipes..38

Dinner Recipes............... 56

Snacks Recipes.................................70

1. Cabbage Apple Stir-Fry
2. Parmesan Roasted Cauliflowe
3. Celery and Fennel Salad with Cranberries
4. Kale with Caramelized Onions
5. Italian- Inspired Rice and Peas
6. Baked Jicama Fries
7. Double-Boiled Sweet Potatoes
8. Roasted Onion Dip

Soup Recipes.................................87

1. Kidney Beans Taco Soup
2. Squash Green Pea Soup
3. Hominy Posole
4. Crab Corn Chowder
5. Chicken Green Beans Soup
6. Cream of Corn Soup
7. Cabbage Beef Borscht
8. Lemon Pepper Beef Soup

10. Jalapeno Crisp

11. Raspberry Popsicle

Introduction

The renal diet contributes to preventing renal failure. Below is a list of food/nutrients you

should avoid preventing kidney-related problems:

Phosphate: Consumption of phosphate becomes dangerous when kidney failure reaches 80% and goes to the 4th/5th stage of kidney failure. So, it is better to lower your phosphate intake by counting the calories and minerals.

Protein: While on a renal diet, you must be eating 0.75 kg protein each day. Good sources of protein are eggs, milk, cheese, meat, nuts, and fish.

Potassium: After getting diagnosed, if your results show your potassium level is high in the blood, you should restrict your potassium intake. Baked and fried potatoes are very high in potassium. Leafy greens, fruit juices are high in potassium. You can still enjoy vegetables that are low in potassium.

Sodium: Adding salt is very important in our food, but when you are suffering from kidney problems, you have to omit or minimize your salt intake. Too much sodium intake can trigger high blood pressure and fluid retention in the body. You need to find substitutes that help season your food. Herbs and spices that are extracted from plants are a good option. Using garlic, pepper, mustard can increase the taste of your food without adding any salt. Avoid artificial "salts" that are low in sodium because they are high in potassium, which is also dangerous for kidney health.

Renal diets help people with kidney disease increase their quality of life.

Other types of food may be harmful to kidneys infected with a disease, so you need to make sure you have a sound knowledge of the infection and how it affects the body.

You don't want kidney disease, but there are ways to boost your well-being by changing your diet. In reality, renal diets help you manage your health and reduce kidney disease.

You need to remember—changing your diet won't heal everybody, but it can help everyone. It doesn't mean a diet is a cure-all, so don't think of this article as medical advice; it's more of a guide.

Your doctor can provide more guidance than this does and should always be informed of any improvement in your condition.

If you have kidney problems, it's essential to regulate your health to help you feel better. There are entire books devoted to renal diets, or you can check with a registered dietitian for recommendations. Using a Kindle or iPad, you can even download and access these books instantly.

Dietitians have experience working with those with kidney problems and can give some general do's and don'ts to follow, such as control potassium intake—fruits like strawberries and apples are low in potassium with vegetables like cauliflower, cabbage, and broccoli.

Track your phosphorous consumption—-creamers, pasta, cereals, and rice are on the OK list.

Restrict liquid intake to 48 oz. Each day's recommended fluid level for renal diets is certain fluid in items like grapes, ice cream, oranges, etc.

Track your salt intake—you'll need to be a tag reader to make sure you keep your salt intake low—know what you're putting in your body and what it might contain.

Regulate your protein intake—maintain 5-7 ounces. Use egg replacements instead of regular eggs as a useful technique for low protein consumption.

If you choose to use a dietitian, they can point you precisely to what you should and shouldn't consume and why. Being aware of the effect food has on your body is essential and can help you feel good every day. Also, this design is not an alternative to clinical guidelines. Yet renal diets help most kidney disease sufferers to become and stay healthier.

Breakfast Recipes

Apple and Cinnamon French Toast Strata

Preparation Time: 2 Hours and 20 Minutes

Cooking Time: 50 Minutes

Servings: 12

Ingredients:

- 1 ½ medium apples peeled, cored, diced

- 1-pound cinnamon and raisin loaf, diced

- One teaspoon ground cinnamon

- ¼ cup pancake syrup

- Six tablespoons unsalted butter, melted

- One ¼ cup half-and-half creamer

- 8 ounces cream cheese, softened and cubed

- Eight large eggs

- One ¼ cup almond milk, unsweetened

Directions:

1. Take a nine 13 inches baking bowl, grease it with oil, then arrange half of the bread cubes on the bottom and scatter cream cheese evenly on the top.

2. Top cream cheese with the apple, sprinkle with cinnamon and then top with remaining bread cubes.

12

3. Crack eggs in a large bowl, add pancake syrup, butter, milk, and creamer, whisk until combined, pour this mixture evenly in the prepared casserole, cover it with plastic wrap, and then keep the casserole dish in the refrigerator for 2 hours.

4. When ready to cook, switch on the oven, set it to 325°F, and preheat.

5. Then uncover casserole, bake for 50 minutes and when done, let it cool for 10 minutes and cut it into twelve three by 3-inches squares.

Drizzle with more pancake syrup and then serve.

Nutrition:

Calories: 324

Fat: 20 g

Protein: 9 g

Carbohydrates: 27 g

Fiber: 1.8 g

Apple and Onion Omelet

Preparation Time: 10 Minutes

Cooking Time: 20 Minutes

Servings: 2

Ingredients:

- One large apple peeled, cored, sliced

- ¾ cup sweet onion, sliced

- One tablespoon unsalted butter

- 1/8 teaspoon ground black pepper

- One tablespoon water

- ¼ cup milk, low-fat

- Two tablespoons shredded cheddar cheese, low-fat

- Three eggs

Directions:

1. Switch on the oven, then set it to 400°F and let it preheat.

2. Crack eggs in a bowl, add black pepper and water, and whisk until beaten.

3. Take a small heatproof skillet pan, place it over medium heat, add butter and when it melts, add onions and apple and cook for 6 minutes until sautéed.

4. Spread onion-apple mixture evenly, pour egg mixture over it, spread evenly, and cook for 2 minutes until eggs begin to set.

5. Then sprinkle cheese on top of eggs, transfer skillet pan into the heated oven, and bake for 12 minutes or until omelet has set.

6. When done, remove the pan from the oven, cut the omelet in half, distribute it between two plates, and then serve.

Nutrition:

Calories: 282

Fat: 16 g

Protein: 13 g

Carbohydrates: 22 g

Fiber: 3.5 g

Asparagus and Cauliflower Tortilla

Preparation Time: 10 Minutes

Cooking Time: 25 Minutes

Servings: 4

Ingredients:

- 2 cups asparagus, chopped and trimmed
- 1 ½ cups white onion, chopped
- 2 cups cauliflower florets, chopped
- ½ teaspoon minced garlic
- ¼ teaspoon ground nutmeg
- ½ teaspoon ground black pepper
- ¼ teaspoon salt
- ¼ teaspoon dried thyme leaves
- Two tablespoons parsley, chopped
- Two teaspoons olive oil
- 1 cup liquid egg substitute, low-cholesterol
- One tablespoon water

Directions:

1. Take a heatproof bowl, add cauliflower florets and asparagus,

drizzle with water, cover the bowl with plastic wrap, pierce

some holes in it, and microwave for 5 minutes, or until tendercrisp.

2. Meanwhile, take a medium-sized skillet pan, place it over

medium heat, add oil, and when hot, add onion and cook for 7

minutes until golden brown.

3. Stir in garlic, cook for 1 minute up until aromatic, switch heat to

medium-low level, add steamed cauliflower-asparagus mixture

in the pan, sprinkle with nutmeg, black pepper, salt, thyme, and

parsley, and pour in egg substitute.

4. Continue cooking for 10 to 15 minutes. You may wait until the

tortilla has set. Wait for the bottom is nicely browned. When

done, slide the tortilla onto a dish. Cut it by running the knife

along the edges.

5. Cut tortilla into four pieces and then serve.

Nutrition:

Calories: 102

Fat: 3 g

Protein: 9 g

Carbohydrates: 9 g

Fiber: 3.8 g

Avocado Toast with Egg

Preparation Time: 10 Minutes

Cooking Time: 5 Minutes

Servings: 2 Toasts

Ingredients:

- ½ of a medium avocado, pitted and sliced

- One tablespoon parsley, chopped

- ¼ teaspoon ground black pepper

- 1/8 teaspoon salt

- One tablespoon lime juice

- Two tablespoons feta cheese, crumbled

- Two eggs

- Two slices of whole-grain bread, toasted

Directions:

1. Transfer avocado flesh to a medium bowl, mash with a fork and then stir in salt and lime juice.

2. Spread the avocado mixture evenly onto each piece of toast, then take a skillet pan, spray it with oil and hot, crack eggs into it and cook to the desired level.

3. Distribute eggs onto the toast, top each piece of toast with ½

tablespoon parsley, one tablespoon cheese, and 1/8 teaspoon ground black pepper.

4. Serve straight away.

Nutrition:

Calories: 225

Fat: 13 g

Protein: 12 g

Carbohydrates:15 g

Fiber: 4.3 g

Baked Egg Cups

Preparation Time: 20 Minutes

Cooking Time: 35 Minutes

Servings: 12 Muffins

Ingredients:

- 1/3 cup mushrooms, diced

- ¼ teaspoon ground black pepper

- 1/3 cup green bell pepper, diced

- 1/3 cup white onion, diced

- Six slices bacon, low-sodium

- 12 eggs

Directions:

1. Switch on the oven, then set it to 350°F and let it preheat.

2. Meanwhile, take a twelve-cup muffin tray, line it with muffin liners, and set aside until required.

3. Take a medium-sized skillet pan, place it over medium heat.

4. When hot, add bacon slices and cook for 7 to 10 minutes, or until crispy.

5. When the bacon has cooked, transfer it to a cutting board, let it cool for 5 minutes, chop the bacon, and then transfer it to a

bowl.

6. Add all the vegetables in the bowl containing bacon, stir until well mixed, and then distribute the mixture evenly between prepared muffin cups.

7. Take another bowl, crack eggs in it, add black pepper, whisk until combined, pour this mixture evenly into muffin cups, and bake into the heated oven for 25 minutes, or until firm and when the tops are golden brown.

8. When done, let muffins cool for 5 minutes, then take them out, let the muffins cool for an additional 10 minutes, and serve.

Nutrition:

Calories: 80

Fat: 5 g

Protein: 7 g

Carbohydrates: 1 g

Fiber: 0.1 g

Breakfast Burrito

Preparation Time: 10 Minutes

Cooking Time: 3 Minutes

Servings: 2

Ingredients:

- Three tablespoons green chiles, diced
- ½ teaspoon hot pepper sauce
- ¼ teaspoon ground cumin
- Four eggs
- Two flour tortillas, burrito size

Directions:

1. Take a medium-sized skillet pan, place it over medium heat, grease it with oil, and let it get hot.

2. Crack eggs in a bowl, add chilies, hot sauce, and cumin, whisk until combined, then pour the egg mixture in the hot skillet, cook for 2 minutes, or until eggs have been cooked to the desired level.

3. Meanwhile, heat the tortillas by microwaving them for 20 seconds until hot.

4. When eggs have cooked, distribute evenly between hot tortillas

and roll it up like a burrito.

5. Serve straight away.

Nutrition:

Calories: 366

Fat: 18 g

Protein: 18 g

Carbohydrates: 33 g

Fiber: 2.5 g

Chorizo and Egg Tortilla

Preparation Time: 10 Minutes

Cooking Time: 13 Minutes

Servings: 1

Ingredients:

- One flour tortilla, about 6-inches

- 1/3 cup chorizo meat, chopped

- One egg

Directions:

1. Take a formed-sized skillet pan, place it over medium heat, add chorizo, and cook for 5 to 8 minutes until done.

2. When the meat has cooked, drain the excess fat, whisk an egg, pour it into the pan, stir until combined, and cook for 3 minutes, or until eggs have cooked.

Spoon egg onto the tortilla and then serve.

Nutrition:

Calories: 223

Fat: 11 g

Protein: 16 g

Carbohydrates: 15 g

Fiber: 1.5 g

Cottage Cheese Pancakes

Preparation Time: 10 Minutes

Cooking Time: 50 Minutes

Servings: 6

Ingredients:

- 3 cups fresh raspberries, sliced
- ½ cup all-purpose white flour
- 1 cup cottage cheese, softened
- Six tablespoons unsalted butter, melted
- Four eggs, beaten

Directions:

1. Crack eggs in a medium-sized bowl, add flour, cheese, and butter it, and whisk until combined.

2. Take a medium-high frying pan, grease it with oil and when hot, pour in prepared batter, ¼ cup of batter per pancake, spread the batter into a 4-inch pancake, and cook for 3 minutes per side until browned.

3. When done, transfer pancakes onto a plate, cook more pancakes in the same manner, and, when done, serve each pancake with ½ sliced raspberries.

Nutrition:

Calories: 253

Fat: 17 g

Protein: 11 g

Carbohydrates: 21 g

Fiber: 2 g

Egg in a Hole

Preparation Time: 5 Minutes

Cooking Time: 5 Minutes

Servings: 1

Ingredients:

One slice of white bread

¼ teaspoon lemon pepper seasoning, salt-free

One egg

One teaspoon Parmesan cheese, grated

Directions:

1. Prepare the bread by making a hole in the middle: use a cookie cutter for cutting out the center.

2. Brush the slice with oil on both sides, then take a medium-sized skillet pan, place it over medium heat and when hot, add bread slice in it, crack the egg in the center of the slice sprinkle with lemon pepper seasoning.

3. Cook the egg for 2 minutes, then carefully flip it along with the slice and continue cooking for an additional 2 minutes.

4. Sprinkle cheese on the egg, let it melt, slide the egg onto a plate, serve straight away.

Nutrition:

Calories: 159

Fat: 7 g

Protein: 9 g

Carbohydrates: 15 g

Fiber: 0.8 g

German Pancakes

Preparation Time: 10 Minutes

Cooking Time: 15 Minutes

Servings: 10

Ingredients:

- 2/3 cup all-purpose flour

- ¼ teaspoon vanilla extract, unsweetened

- Two tablespoons white sugar

- 1 cup milk, low-fat

- Four eggs

- One ¼ cup cream cheese softened

- 1/3 cup fruit jam for serving, sugar-free

Directions:

1. Prepare the batter by taking a medium-sized bowl, add flour in it along with sugar, stir until mixed, whisk in eggs until blended, and then whisk in vanilla and milk until smooth.

2. Take a skillet pan, about 8 inches, spray it with oil and when hot, add three tablespoons of the prepared batter, tilt the pan to spread the batter evenly, and cook for 45 seconds, or until the bottom is browned.

3. Flip the pancake, continue cooking for 45 seconds until the other side is browned, and when done, transfer pancake to a plate.

4. Cook nine more pancakes in the same manner and, when done, spread two tablespoons of cream cheese on one side of the pancake, fold it, and then serve with one tablespoon of fruit jam.

Nutrition:

Calories: 74

Fat: 2 g

Protein: 4 g

Carbohydrates: 10 g

Fiber: 0.2 g

Mushroom and Red Pepper Omelet

Preparation Time: 5 Minutes

Cooking Time: 12 Minutes

Servings: 2

Ingredients:

- Two tablespoons white onion, diced

- ¼ cup sweet red peppers, diced

- ½ cup mushrooms, diced

- ¼ teaspoon ground black pepper

- One teaspoon Worcestershire sauce

- Two teaspoons unsalted butter

- Three eggs

- Two tablespoons whipped cream cheese

Directions:

1. Take a medium-sized skillet pan, place it over medium heat, add one teaspoon butter and when it melts, add onions and mushrooms and cook for 5 minutes, or until onions are tender.

2. Stir in red pepper, then transfer vegetables to a plate and set aside until needed.

3. Crack the eggs in a bowl, add Worcestershire sauce, and whisk

until combined.

4. Return skillet pan over medium heat, add remaining butter, and when it melts, pour in the egg mixture, and cook for 2 minutes or until omelet is partially cooked.

5. Then top cooked vegetables on one side of the omelet, top with cream cheese, and continue cooking until omelet is cooked thoroughly.

6. When done, take away the pan from the heat, cover the omelet's filling by folding the other half of the omelet, sprinkle it with black pepper, and then divide it into two.

7. Serve straight away.

Nutrition:

Calories: 199

Fat: 15 g

Protein: 11 g

Carbohydrates: 4 g

Fiber: 0.6 g

Blueberry Blast Smoothie

Preparation Time: 10 Minutes

Cooking Time: 0 Minutes

Servings: 1

Ingredients:

- 1 cup frozen blueberries

- Eight packets of Splenda

- 6 tbsp of protein powder

- Eight ice cubes

- 14 oz apple juice

Directions:

1. First, start by hitting all the ingredients in a blender jug.

2. Give it a pulse for 30 seconds until blended well.

3. Serve chilled and fresh.

Nutrition:

Calories 108 Protein 9 g Fat 0.2 g Cholesterol 0.01 mg

Potassium 183 mg Calcium 57mgb Fiber 1.2g

Pineapple Protein Smoothie

Preparation Time: 10 Minutes

Cooking Time: 0 Minutes

Servings: 1

Ingredients:

- 3/4 cup pineapple sorbet

- One scoop vanilla protein powder

- 1/2 cup water

- Two ice cubes, optional

Directions:

1. First, start by putting all the fixings in a blender jug.

2. Give it a pulse for 30 seconds until blended well.

3. Serve chilled and fresh.

Nutrition:

Calories 268

Protein 18 g

Fat 4g

Cholesterol 36 mg

Potassium 237 mg Calcium 160 mg

Fiber 1.4g

Fruity Smoothie

Preparation Time: 10 Minutes

Cooking Time: 0 Minutes

Servings: 2

Ingredients:

- 8 oz canned fruits, with juice

- Two scoops of vanilla-flavored whey protein powder

- 1 cup of cold water

- 1 cup crushed ice

Directions:

1. First, start by putting all the fixings in a blender jug.

2. Give it a pulse for 30 seconds until blended well.

3. Serve chilled and fresh.

Nutrition:

Calories 186

Protein 23 g

Fat 2g

Cholesterol 41 mg

Potassium 282 mg

Calcium 160 mg Fiber 1.1 g

Mixed Berry Protein Smoothie

Preparation Time: 10 Minutes

Cooking Time: 0 Minutes

Servings: 2

Ingredients:

- 4 oz cold water

- 1 cup of frozen mixed berries

- Two ice cubes

- 1 tsp blueberry essence

- 1/2 cup whipped cream topping

- Two scoops of whey protein powder

Directions:

1. First, start by putting all the fixings in a blender jug.

2. Give it a pulse for 30 seconds until blended well.

3. Serve chilled and fresh.

Nutrition: Calories 104 Protein 6 g Fat 4 g Cholesterol 11 mg Potassium 141 mg Calcium 69 mg Fiber 2.4 g

Lunch Recipes

Shrimp Paella

Preparation Time: 5 Minutes

Cooking Time: 10 Minutes

Servings: 2

Ingredients:

- 1 cup cooked brown rice
- One chopped red onion
- 1 tsp. paprika
- One chopped garlic clove
- 1 tbsp. olive oil
- 6 oz. frozen cooked shrimp
- One deseeded and sliced chili pepper
- 1 tbsp. oregano

Directions:

1. Warm the olive oil in a pan on medium-high heat.

2. Add the onion and garlic and sauté for 2-3 minutes until soft.

3. Now add the shrimp and sauté for a further 5 minutes or until hot through.

4. Now add the herbs, spices, chili, and rice with 1/2 cup boiling water.

5. Stir until everything is warm, and the water has been absorbed.

6. Plate up and serve.

Nutrition:

Calories 221

Protein 17 g

Carbs 31 g

Fat 8 g

Sodium (Na) 235 mg

Potassium (K) 176 mg

Phosphorus 189 mg

Salmon and Pesto Salad

Preparation Time: 5 Minutes

Cooking Time: 15 Minutes

Servings: 2

Ingredients:

For the pesto:

- One minced garlic clove
- ½ cup fresh arugula
- ¼ cup extra virgin olive oil
- ½ cup fresh basil
- 1 tsp. black pepper

For the salmon:

- 4 oz. skinless salmon fillet
- 1 tbsp. coconut oil

For the salad:

- ½ juiced lemon

- Two sliced radishes
- ½ cup iceberg lettuce
- 1 tsp. black pepper

Directions:

1. Prepare the pesto by blending all the pesto ingredients in a food processor or grinding with a pestle and mortar. Set aside.

2. Add a skillet to the stove on medium-high heat and melt the coconut oil.

3. Add the salmon to the pan.

4. Cook for 7-8 minutes and turn over.

5. Cook for an additional 3-4 minutes or up until cooked through.

6. Remove fillets from the skillet and allow to rest.

7. Mix the lettuce and the radishes and squeeze over the juice of ½ lemon.

8. Flake the salmon with a fork and mix through the salad.

9. Toss to coat and sprinkle with a little black pepper to serve.

Nutrition:

Calories 221

Protein 13 g

Carbs 1 g

Fat 34 g

Sodium (Na) 80 mg

Potassium (K) 119 mg

Phosphorus 158 mg

Baked Fennel and Garlic Sea Bass

Preparation Time: 5 Minutes

Cooking Time: 15 Minutes

Servings: 2

Ingredients:

- One lemon
- ½ sliced fennel bulb
- 6 oz. sea bass fillets
- 1 tsp. black pepper
- Two garlic cloves

Directions:

1. Preheat the oven to 375°F/Gas Spot 5.

2. Sprinkle black pepper over the Sea Bass.

3. Slice the fennel bulb and garlic cloves.

4. Add one salmon fillet and half the fennel and garlic to one sheet of baking paper or tin foil.

5. Squeeze in 1/2 lemon juices.

6. Repeat for the other fillet.

7. Fold and add to the oven for 12-15 minutes or until fish is thoroughly cooked through.

8. Meanwhile, add boiling water to your couscous, cover, and allow to steam.

9. Serve with your choice of rice or salad.

Nutrition: Calories 221

Protein 14 g Carbs 3 g Fat 2 g Sodium (Na) 119 mg Potassium (K) 398 mg Phosphorus 149 mg

Lemon, Garlic & Cilantro Tuna and Rice

Preparation Time: 5 Minutes

Cooking Time: 0 Minutes

Servings: 2

Ingredients:

- ½ cup arugula
- 1 tbsp. extra virgin olive oil
- 1 cup cooked rice
- 1 tsp. black pepper
- ¼ finely diced red onion
- One juiced lemon
- 3 oz. canned tuna
- 2 tbsps. Chopped fresh cilantro

Directions:

1. Mix the olive oil, pepper, cilantro, and red onion in a bowl.

2. Stir in the tuna, cover, and leave in the fridge for as long as possible. Serve immediately.

3. When ready to eat, serve up with the cooked rice and arugula!

Nutrition:

Calories 221

Protein 11 g

Carbs 26 g

Fat 7 g

Sodium (Na) 143 mg

Potassium (K)197 mgPhosphorus 182 mg

Cod & Green Bean Risotto

Preparation Time: 4 Minutes

Cooking Time: 40 Minutes

Servings: 2

Ingredients:

- ½ cup arugula
- One finely diced white onion
- 4 oz. cod fillet
- 1 cup white rice
- Two lemon wedges
- 1 cup boiling water
- ¼ tsp. black pepper
- 1 cup low sodium chicken broth
- 1 tbsp. extra virgin olive oil
- ½ cup green beans

Directions:

1. Heat the oil in a large pan on standard heat.

2. Sauté the chopped onion for 5 minutes until soft before adding in the rice and stirring for 1-2 minutes.

3. Combine the broth with boiling water.

4. Add half of the liquid to the pan and stir slowly.

5. Slowly add the rest of the liquid while continuously stirring for up to 20-30 minutes.

6. Stir in the green beans to the risotto.

7. Place the fish on top of the rice, cover, and steam for 10

minutes.

8. Ensure the water does not dry out and keep topping up until the rice is cooked thoroughly.

9. Use your fork to break up the fish fillets and stir into the rice.

10. Sprinkle with freshly ground pepper to serve and a squeeze of fresh lemon.

11. Garnish with the lemon wedges and serve with the arugula.

Nutrition:

Calories 221

Protein 12 g

Carbs 29 g

Fat 8 g

Sodium (Na) 398 mg

Potassium (K) 347 mg

Phosphorus 241 mg

Mixed Pepper Stuffed River Trout

Preparation Time: 5 Minutes

Cooking Time: 20 Minutes

Servings: 4

Ingredients:

One whole river trout

- 1 tsp. thyme
- ¼ diced yellow pepper
- 1 cup baby spinach leaves
- ¼ diced green pepper
- One juiced lime
- ¼ diced red pepper
- 1 tsp. oregano
- 1 tsp. extra virgin olive oil
- 1 tsp. black pepper

Directions:

1. Preheat the broiler /grill on high heat.

2. Lightly oil a baking tray.

3. Mix all of the fixings apart from the trout and lime.

4. Slice the trout lengthways (there should be an opening here from where it was gutted) and stuff the mixed ingredients inside.

5. Squeeze the lime juice over the fish and then place the lime wedges on the tray.

6. Place under the broiler on the baking tray and broil for 15-20

minutes or until fish is thoroughly cooked through and flakes easily.

7. Enjoy alone or with a side helping of rice or salad.

Nutrition: Calories 290 Protein 15 g Carbs 0 g Fat 7 g Sodium (Na)43 mg Potassium (K) 315 mg Phosphorus 189 mg

Haddock & Buttered Leeks

Preparation Time: 5 Minutes

Cooking Time: 15 Minutes

Servings: 2

Ingredients:

- 1 tbsp. unsalted butter
- One sliced leek
- ¼ tsp. black pepper
- 2 tsp. Chopped parsley
- 6 oz. haddock fillets
- ½ juiced lemon

Directions:

1. Preheat the oven to 375°F/Gas Mark 5.

2. Add the haddock fillets to baking or parchment paper and sprinkle with the black pepper.

3. Squeeze over the lemon juice and wrap into a parcel.

4. Bake the parcel on a baking tray for 10-15 minutes or until the fish is thoroughly cooked through.

5. Meanwhile, heat the butter over medium-low heat in a small pan.

6. Add the leeks and parsley and sauté for 5-7 minutes until soft.

7. Serve the haddock fillets on a bed of buttered leeks and enjoy!

Nutrition: Calories 124 Protein 15 g Carbs 0 g Fat 7 g Sodium (Na) 161 mg Potassium (K) 251 mg Phosphorus 220 mg

Thai Spiced Halibut

Preparation Time: 5 Minutes

Cooking Time: 20 Minutes

Servings: 2

Ingredients:

- 2 tbsps. coconut oil
- 1 cup white rice
- ¼ tsp. black pepper
- ½ diced red chili
- 1 tbsp. fresh basil
- 2 pressed garlic cloves
- 4 oz. halibut fillet
- One halved lime
- Two sliced green onions
- One lime leaf

Directions:

1. Preheat oven to 400°F/Gas Mark 5.

2. Add half of the ingredients into baking paper and fold into a parcel.

3. Repeat for your second parcel.

4. Add to the oven for 15-20 minutes or until fish is thoroughly cooked through.

5. Serve with cooked rice.

Nutrition:

Calories 311

Protein 16 g

Carbs 17 g

Fat 15 g

Sodium (Na) 31 mg

Potassium (K) 418 mg

Phosphorus 257 mg

Homemade Tuna Niçoise

Preparation Time: 5 Minutes

Cooking Time: 10 Minutes

Servings: 2

Ingredients:

- One egg
- ½ cup green beans
- ¼ sliced cucumber
- One juiced lemon
- 1 tsp. black pepper
- ¼ sliced red onion
- 1 tbsp. olive oil
- 1 tbsp. capers
- 4 oz. drained canned tuna
- Four iceberg lettuce leaves
- 1 tsp. chopped fresh cilantro

Directions:

1. Prepare the salad by washing and slicing the lettuce, cucumber, and onion.

2. Add to a salad bowl.

3. Mix 1 tbsp oil with the lemon juice, cilantro, and capers for a salad dressing. Set aside.

4. Boil a pan of water on high heat, then lower to simmer and add the egg for 6 minutes. (Steam the green beans over the same pan in a steamer/colander for 6 minutes).

5. Remove the egg and rinse under cold water.

6. Peel before slicing in half.

7. Mix the tuna, salad, and dressing together in a salad bowl.

8. Toss to coat.

9. Top with the egg and serve with a sprinkle of black pepper.

Nutrition:

Calories 199

Protein 19 g

Carbs 7 g

Fat 8 g

Sodium (Na) 466 mg

Potassium (K) 251 mg

Phosphorus 211 mg

Monk-Fish Curry

Preparation Time: 5 Minutes

Cooking Time: 20 Minutes

Servings: 2

Ingredients:

- One garlic clove
- Three finely chopped green onions
- 1 tsp. grated ginger
- 1 cup of water.
- 2 tsp. Chopped fresh basil
- 1 cup cooked rice noodles
- 1 tbsp. coconut oil
- ½ sliced red chili
- 4 oz. Monk-fish fillet
- ½ finely sliced stick lemon-grass
- 2 tbsps. chopped shallots

Directions:

1. Slice the monkfish into bite-size pieces.

2. By means of a pestle, also mortar or food processor, crush the basil, garlic, ginger, chili, and lemon-grass to form a paste.

3. Heat the oil in a pan over medium-high heat and add the shallots.

4. Now add the water to the pan and bring to a boil.

5. Add the Monk-fish, lower the heat and cover to simmer for 10 minutes or until cooked through.

6. Enjoy with rice noodles and scatter with green onions to serve.

Nutrition:

Calories 249

Protein 12 g

Carbs 30 g

Fat 10 g

Sodium (Na) 32 mg

Potassium (K) 398 mg

Phosphorus 190 mg

Salad with Vinaigrette

Preparation Time: 25 Minutes

Cooking Time: 0 Minutes

Servings: 4

Ingredients:

- For the vinaigrette
- ½ cup Olive oil
- 4 tbsps balsamic vinegar
- 2 tbsps chopped fresh oregano
- Pinch red pepper flakes
- Ground black pepper
- For the salad
- 4 cups shredded green leaf lettuce
- 1 carrot, shredded
- ¾ cup, cut into 1-inch pieces fresh green beans –
- 3 large radishes, sliced thin

Directions:

1. To make the vinaigrette: put the vinaigrette ingredients in a bowl and whisk.

2. In a bowl, make the salad, pitch together with the carrot, lettuce, green beans, and radishes.

3. Add the vinaigrette to the vegetables and toss to coat.

4. Arrange the salad on plates and serve.

Nutrition: Calories: 273 Fat: 27 g Carb: 7 g Phosphorus: 30 mg Potassium: 197 mg Sodium: 27 mg Protein: 1 g

Dinner Recipes

Roasted Citrus Chicken

Preparation Time: 20 Minutes

Cooking Time: 60 Minutes

Servings: 8

Ingredients:

- 1 tablespoon olive oil
- 2 cloves garlic, minced
- 1 teaspoon Italian seasoning
- ½ teaspoon black pepper
- 8 chicken thighs
- 2 cups chicken broth, reduced-sodium
- 3 tablespoons lemon juice
- ½ large chicken breast for one chicken thigh

Directions:

1. Warm oil in the considerable skillet.

2. Include garlic and seasonings.

3. Include chicken bosoms and dark-colored all sides.

4. Spot chicken in the moderate cooker and include the chicken soup.

5. Cook on LOW heat for 6 to 8hours

6. Include lemon juice toward the part of the bargain time.

Nutrition:

Calories: 265

Fat: 19 g

Protein: 21 gCarbs: 1 g

Chicken with Asian Vegetables

Preparation Time: 10 Minutes

Cooking Time: 20 Minutes

Servings: 8

Ingredients:

- 2 tablespoons canola oil
- 6 boneless chicken breasts
- 1 cup low-sodium chicken broth
- 3 tablespoons reduced-sodium soy sauce
- ¼ teaspoon crushed red pepper flakes
- 1 garlic clove, crushed
- 1 can (8ounces) water chestnuts, sliced and rinsed (optional)
- ½ cup sliced green onions
- 1 cup chopped red or green bell pepper
- 1 cup chopped celery
- ¼ cup cornstarch
- 1/3 cup water
- 3 cups cooked white rice
- ½ large chicken breast for one chicken thigh

Directions:

1. Warm oil in a skillet and dark-colored chicken on all sides.

2. Add chicken to a slow cooker with the remainder of the fixings aside from cornstarch and water.

3. Spread and cook on LOW for 6 to 8hours

4. Following 6-8 hours, independently blend cornstarch and cold

58

water until smooth. Gradually include into the moderate cooker.

5. At that point, turn on high for about 15mins until thickened. Don't close the top on the moderate cooker to enable steam to leave.

6. Serve Asian blend over rice.

Nutrition:

Calories: 415

Fat: 20 g

Protein: 20 g

Carbs: 36 g

Chicken Adobo

Preparation Time: 10 Minutes

Cooking Time: 40 Minutes

Servings: 6

Ingredients:

- 4 medium yellow onions, halved and thinly sliced
- 4 medium garlic cloves, smashed and peeled
- 1 (5-inch) piece fresh ginger, cut into
- 1 inch pieces
- 1 bay leaf
- 3 pounds bone-in chicken thighs
- 3 tablespoons reduced-sodium soy sauce
- ¼ cup rice vinegar (not seasoned)
- 1 tablespoon granulated sugar
- ½ teaspoon freshly ground black pepper

Directions:

1. Spot the onions, garlic, ginger, and narrows leaf in an even layer in the small cooker.

2. Take out and do away with the pores and skin from the chicken.

3. Organize the hen in an even layer over the onion mixture.

4. Beat the soy sauce, vinegar, sugar, and pepper collectively in a medium bowl and pour it over the fowl.

5. Spread and prepare dinner on LOW for 8hours

6. Evacuate and take away the ginger portions and inlet leaves.

7. Present with steamed rice.

Nutrition:

Calories: 318

Fat: 9 g

Protein: 14 g

Carbs: 44 g

Chicken and Veggie Soup

Preparation Time: 15 Minutes

Cooking Time: 25 Minutes

Servings: 8

Ingredients:

- 4 cups cooked and chopped chicken
- 7 cups reduced-sodium chicken broth
- 1 pound froze white corn
- 1 medium onion diced
- 4 cloves garlic minced
- 2 carrots peeled and diced
- 2 celery stalks chopped
- 2 teaspoons oregano
- 2 teaspoon curry powder
- ½ teaspoon black pepper

Directions:

1. Include all fixings into the moderate cooker.

2. Cook on LOW for 8hours

3. Serve over cooked white rice.

Nutrition:

Calories: 220

Fat:7 g

Protein: 24 g

Carbs: 19 g

Turkey Sausages

Preparation Time: 10 Minutes

Cooking Time: 10 Minutes

Servings: 2

Ingredients:

- 1/4 teaspoon salt
- 1/8 teaspoon garlic powder
- 1/8 teaspoon onion powder
- One teaspoon fennel seed
- 1 pound 7% fat ground turkey

Directions:

1. Press the fennel seed and put together turkey with fennel seed, garlic, onion powder, and salt in a small cup.

2. Cover the bowl and refrigerate overnight.

3. Prepare the turkey with seasoning into different portions with a circle form and press them into patties ready to be cooked.

4. Cook at medium heat until browned.

5. Cook it for 1 to 2 minutes per side and serve them hot. Enjoy!

Nutrition:

Calories: 55

Protein: 7 g

Sodium: 70 mg

Potassium: 105 mg

Phosphorus: 75 mg

Rosemary Chicken

Preparation Time: 10 Minutes

Cooking Time: 10 Minutes

Servings: 2

Ingredients:

- Two zucchinis
- One carrot
- One teaspoon dried rosemary
- Four chicken breasts
- 1/2 bell pepper
- 1/2 red onion
- Eight garlic cloves
- Olive oil
- 1/4 tablespoon ground pepper

Directions:

1. Prepare the oven and preheat it at 375 °F (or 200°C).

2. Slice both zucchini and carrots and add bell pepper, onion, garlic, and put everything adding oil in a 13" x 9" pan.

3. Spread the pepper over everything and roast for about 10 minutes.

4. Meanwhile, lift the chicken skin and spread black pepper and rosemary on the flesh.

5. Take away the vegetable pan from the oven and add the chicken, returning it to the oven for about 30 more minutes.

Serve and enjoy!

Nutrition:

Calories: 215

Protein: 28 g

Sodium: 105 mg

Potassium: 580 mg

Phosphorus: 250 mg

Smokey Turkey Chili

Preparation Time: 5 Minutes

Cooking Time: 45 Minutes

Servings: 8

Ingredients:

- 12ounce lean ground turkey
- 1/2 red onion, chopped
- Two cloves garlic, crushed and chopped
- ½ teaspoon of smoked paprika
- ½ teaspoon of chili powder
- ½ teaspoon of dried thyme
- ¼ cup reduced-sodium beef stock
- ½ cup of water
- 1 ½ cups baby spinach leaves, washed
- Three wheat tortillas

Directions:

1. Brown the ground beef in a dry skillet over medium-high heat.

2. Add in the red onion and garlic.

3. Sauté the onion until it goes clear.

4. Transfer the contents of the skillet to the slow cooker.

5. Add the remaining ingredients and simmer on low for 30–45 minutes.

6. Stir through the spinach for the last few minutes to wilt.

7. Slice tortillas and gently toast under the broiler until slightly crispy.

8. Serve on top of the turkey chili.

Nutrition:

Calories: 93.5

Protein: 8g

Carbohydrates: 3 g

Fat: 5.5 g

Cholesterol: 30.5 mg

Sodium: 84.5 mg

Potassium: 142.5 mg

Fiber: 0.5 g

Avocado-Orange Grilled Chicken

Preparation Time: 20 Minutes

Cooking Time: 60 Minutes

Servings: 4

Ingredients:

- ¼ cup fresh lime juice
- ¼ cup minced red onion
- One avocado
- 1 cup low-fat yogurt
- One small red onion, sliced thinly
- One tablespoon honey
- Two oranges, peeled and cut
- Two tablespoons. chopped cilantro
- Four pieces of 4-6ounce boneless, skinless chicken breasts
- Pepper and salt to taste

Directions:

1. In a large bowl, mix honey, cilantro, minced red onion, and yogurt.

2. Submerge chicken into mixture and marinate for at least 30 minutes.

3. Grease grate and preheat grill to medium-high fire.

4. Remove chicken from marinade and season with pepper and salt.

5. Grill for 6 minutes per side or until chicken is cooked and juices run clear.

6. Meanwhile, peel the avocado and discard the seed—chop avocados and place in a bowl. Quickly add lime juice and toss avocado to coat well with liquid.

7. Add cilantro, thinly sliced onions, and oranges into the bowl of avocado, mix well.

8. Serve grilled chicken and avocado dressing on the side.

Nutrition:

Calories per Serving: 209

Carbs: 26 g

Protein: 8 g

Fats: 10 g

Phosphorus: 157 mg

Potassium: 548 mg

Sodium: 125 mg

Snacks Recipes

Cabbage Apple Stir-Fry

Preparation Time: 15 Minutes

Cooking Time: 10 Minutes

Servings: 4

Ingredients:

- Two tablespoons extra-virgin olive oil

- 3 cups chopped red cabbage

- Two tablespoons water

- 1 Granny Smith apple, chopped

- Three scallions, both white and green parts, chopped

- One tablespoon freshly squeezed lemon juice

- One teaspoon caraway seed

- Pinch salt

Directions:

1. In a big skillet or frying pan, heat the olive oil over medium-high temperature.

2. Add the cabbage and stir-fry for 2 minutes. Add the water, cover, and cook for 2 minutes.

3. Uncover and stir in the apple and scallions and sprinkle with the lemon juice, caraway seeds, and salt—Stir-fry for 4 to 6

minutes longer, or until the cabbage is crisp-tender. Serve.

Nutrition:

Calories: 106

Total fat: 7 g

Saturated fat: 1 g

Sodium: 55 mg

Phosphorus: 27 mg

Potassium: 206 mg

Carbohydrates: 11 g

Fiber: 3 g

Protein: 1 g

Sugar: 7 g

Parmesan Roasted Cauliflower

Preparation Time: 15 Minutes

Cooking Time: 25 Minutes

Servings: 4

Ingredients:

- 4 cups cauliflower florets

- ½ cup grated Parmesan cheese

- Two tablespoons extra-virgin olive oil

- Four garlic cloves, minced

- ½ teaspoon dried thyme leaves

- ¼ teaspoon freshly ground black pepper

- 1/8 teaspoon salt

Directions:

1. Preheat the oven to 400°F.

2. On a baking sheet, combine the cauliflower, Parmesan cheese, olive oil, garlic, thyme, pepper, salt, and toss to coat.

3. Bake for 25 to 30 minutes, stirring once during the cooking time until the cauliflower has light golden-brown edges and is tender. Serve.

Nutrition:

Calories: 144

Total fat: 11 g

Saturated fat: 3 g

Sodium: 332 mg

Phosphorus: 130 mg

Potassium: 359 mg

Carbohydrates: 4 g

Fiber: 1 g

Protein: 6 g

Sugar: 2 g

Celery and Fennel Salad with Cranberries

Preparation Time: 15 Minutes

Cooking Time: 0 Minutes

Servings: 6

Ingredients:

- ¼ cup extra-virgin olive oil

- Two tablespoons freshly squeezed lemon juice

- One tablespoon Dijon mustard

- 2 cups sliced celery

- ½ cup chopped fennel

- ½ cup dried cranberries

- Two tablespoons minced celery leaves

Directions:

1. In a serving bowl, paddle the olive oil, lemon juice, and mustard.

2. Add the celery, fennel, and cranberries to the dressing and toss to coat. Sprinkle with the celery leaves and serve.

Nutrition:

Calories: 130

Total fat: 9 g

Sodium: 88 mg

Phosphorus: 13 mg

Potassium: 107 mg

Carbohydrates: 13 g

Fiber: 1 g

Protein: <1 g

Sugar: 10 g

Kale with Caramelized Onions

Preparation Time: 15 Minutes

Cooking Time: 20 Minutes

Servings: 4

Ingredients:

- One yellow onion, chopped

- Two tablespoons butter

- One tablespoon extra-virgin olive oil

- One bunch kale, rinsed and torn into pieces

- Two tablespoons water

- One tablespoon freshly squeezed lemon juice

- One teaspoon maple syrup

- Salt

- Freshly ground black pepper

Directions:

1. In a heavy saucepan, combine the onion, butter, and olive oil over medium heat. Cook for about 3 minutes, until the onion starts to become translucent, stirring frequently.

2. Reduce the heat to low and continue cooking for 10 to 15 minutes longer, frequently stirring, until the onion starts to

brown.

3. Surge the heat to medium and add the kale and water. Cover the pan and cook for about 2 minutes, shaking the pan occasionally, until the kale starts to soften.

4. Add the lemon juice and maple syrup and season with salt and pepper. Cook for 3 to 4 minutes longer, frequently stirring, until the kale is tender. Serve.

Nutrition:

Calories: 115

Total fat: 10 g

Saturated fat: 4 g

Sodium: 112 mg

Phosphorus: 37 mg

Potassium: 224 mg

Carbohydrates: 6 g

Fiber: 2 g

Protein: 2 g

Sugar: 3 g

Italian- Inspired Rice and Peas

Preparation Time: 10 Minutes

Cooking Time: 35 Minutes

Servings: 4

Ingredients:

- Two tablespoons extra-virgin olive oil

- One onion, chopped

- 1 cup of brown rice

- 1/8 teaspoon salt

- 2 ½ cups water, divided

- 2 cups frozen baby peas

- ¼ teaspoon dried mint leaves

- Two tablespoons grated Parmesan cheese

Directions:

1. In a large saucepan, heat the olive oil over medium heat.

2. Put the onion then cook for 2 to 3 minutes, stirring, until tender.

3. Add the rice and stir until the rice is coated with the oil. Sprinkle with the salt. Add 1 cup of water; cook for 5 to 10 minutes, stirring, until the water is absorbed.

4. Add another ½ cup of water; cook and stir until it's absorbed,

another 5 minutes. Then add the remaining 1 cup of water, cover the pan, and simmer for about 20 minutes, occasionally stirring, until the rice is tender. Using this method will force the rice to omit some starch and make the dish creamier.

5. Mix the peas and mint to the pan. Cook for 3 to 5 minutes, frequently stirring, until the peas are hot and tender.

6. Sprinkle with the cheese and serve.

Nutrition:

Calories: 317

Total fat: 10 g

Saturated fat: 2 g

Sodium: 207 mg

Phosphorus: 237 mg

Potassium: 312 mg

Carbohydrates: 50 g

Fiber: 5 g

Protein: 9 g

Sugar: 6 g

Baked Jicama Fries

Preparation Time: 20 Minutes

Cooking Time: 50 Minutes

Servings: 4

Ingredients:

- 1-pound jicama root

- Two tablespoons butter

- One tablespoon extra-virgin olive oil

- One teaspoon chili powder

- One teaspoon paprika

- ¼ teaspoon salt

- 1/8 teaspoon freshly ground black pepper

- Two tablespoons grated Parmesan cheese

Directions:

1. Peel the jicama and cut into ½-inch slices. Cut the slices into strips, each about 4 inches long.

2. In a large saucepan, place the jicama strips and cover with water. Bring to a boil, then boil for 9 minutes. Drain the jicama well and transfer to a rimmed baking sheet. Pat the strips with a paper towel while waiting for they are dry so that the stripes will

crisp in the oven.

3. Preheat the oven to 400°F.

4. In a small saucepan, melt the butter with the olive oil. Drizzle over the jicama on the baking sheet. Sprinkle with the chili powder, paprika, salt, and pepper and toss to coat. Spread the strips into a single layer.

5. Bake the jicama fries for 40 to 45 minutes or until they are browned and crisp, turning once with a spatula halfway through the cooking time.

6. Sprinkle with the Parmesan cheese and serve.

Nutrition:

Calories: 140

Total fat: 10 g

Saturated fat: 5 g

Sodium: 273 mg

Phosphorus: 45 mg

Potassium: 204 mg

Carbohydrates: 11 g

Fiber: 6 g

Protein: 2 gSugar: 2 g

Double-Boiled Sweet Potatoes

Preparation Time: 20 Minutes

Cooking Time: 25 Minutes

Servings: 4

Ingredients:

- Two large sweet potatoes, peeled and cut into 1-inch cubes

- Two tablespoons extra-virgin olive oil

- Two tablespoons butter

- One red onion, chopped

- ¼ cup half-and-half

- One tablespoon honey

- ¼ teaspoon salt

- 1/8 teaspoon freshly ground black pepper

Directions:

1. In a large saucepan, fill the pot with water to about an inch above the potatoes. Add the sweet potato cubes and bring to a boil. Boil for 10 minutes.

2. Drain the sweet potatoes, discarding the water.

3. In the same saucepan, fill the pot to the same level again. Add the sweet potato cubes and bring to a boil for 10 to 15 minutes,

or until the potatoes are tender.

4. In the meantime, in a large frying pan, heat the olive oil and butter. Add the red onion and cook for 3 to 5 minutes, stirring, until the onion is very tender.

5. Drain the sweet potatoes once more, discarding the water again. Add the sweet potatoes to the skillet along with the halfand-half, honey, salt, and pepper.

6. Pound the potatoes, using an immersion blender or a potato masher, until the desired consistency. Serve.

Nutrition:

Calories: 246

Total fat: 14 g

Saturated fat: 6 g

Sodium: 235 mg

Phosphorus: 62 mg

Potassium: 201 mg

Carbohydrates: 29 g

Fiber: 3 g

Protein: 2 g

Sugar: 13 g

Roasted Onion Dip

Preparation Time: 15 Minutes

Cooking Time: 35 Minutes

Servings: 1 ½ cups

Ingredients:

- One red onion, chopped

- Two tablespoons extra-virgin olive oil

- 1 (8-ounce) package cream cheese

- Two tablespoons mayonnaise (made with avocado oil or olive

- oil)

- One tablespoon freshly squeezed lemon juice

- ½ teaspoon dried thyme leaves

Directions:

1. Preheat the oven to 400°F.

2. On a rimmed baking sheet, combine the onion and olive oil and toss to coat.

3. Roast for 30 to 35 minutes, occasionally stirring, until the onions are soft and golden brown. Don't let them burn. Transfer to a plate and set aside.

4. In a medium bowl, beat the cream cheese, mayonnaise, lemon juice, and thyme leaves. Stir in the onions.

5. You can serve the dip at this point or cover and refrigerate it up to 8 hours before serving.

Nutrition:

Calories: 212

Total fat: 21 g

Saturated fat: 9 g

Sodium: 149 mg

Phosphorus: 47 mg

Potassium: 82 mg

Carbohydrates: 4 g

Protein: 3 g

Sugar: 2 gensure even cooking. To enjoy!

Soups Recipes

Kidney Beans Taco Soup

Preparation Time: 5 Minutes

Cooking Time: 6 Hours

Servings: 6

Ingredients:

- 1 lb. ground beef
- 1 cup onion, chopped
- Two cans of kidney beans
- One can corn
- 1 (15 oz.) can tomato
- 1 (15 oz.) can tomato sauce
- Black pepper, to taste
- 2 1/2 cups water

Directions:

1. Add the beef, onion, beans, and the rest of the ingredients to a slow cooker.

2. Cover the beans-corn mixture and cook for 6 hours at low temperature.

3. Serve warm.

Nutrition:

Calories 228

Total Fat 5.3 g

Saturated Fat 1.9 g

Cholesterol 68 mg

Sodium 261 mg

Carbohydrate 17.6 g

Dietary Fiber 4.8 g

Sugars 3 g

Protein 27.5 g

Calcium 29 mg

Phosphorous 341 mg

Potassium 624 mg

Squash Green Pea Soup

Preparation Time: 5 Minutes

Cooking Time: 50 Minutes

Servings: 7

Ingredients:

5 cups butternut squash, skinned, seeded, and cubed

5 cups low-sodium chicken broth

Topping:

2 cups fresh green peas

Two tablespoons fresh lime juice

Black pepper, to taste

Directions:

1. Begin by warming the broth and squash in the saucepan on moderate heat.

2. Let it simmer for approximately 45 minutes, then add the black pepper, lime juice, and green peas.

3. Cook for another 5 minutes, then allow it to cool.

4. Puree the soup using the handheld blender until smooth.

5. Serve.

Nutrition:

Calories 152

Total Fat 3.7 g

Saturated Fat 0.3 g

Cholesterol 0 mg

Sodium 21 mg

Carbohydrate 31 g

Dietary Fiber 6.3 g

Sugars 6.6 g

Protein 4.2 g

Calcium 156 mg

Phosphorous 126 mg

Potassium 366 mg

Hominy Posole

Preparation Time: 5 Minutes

Cooking Time: 53 Minutes

Servings: 6

Ingredients:

- Two garlic cloves, peeled

- 1 cup boneless pork, diced

- One tablespoon cumin powder

- One onion, chopped

- Two garlic cloves, chopped

- Two tablespoons oil

- 1/2 teaspoon black pepper

- 1/2 teaspoon cayenne

- Two tablespoons chili powder

- 1/4 teaspoon oregano

- 1 (29 oz.) can of White Hominy, drained

- 5 cups pork broth

- 1 cup canned diced green chilis

- Two jalapeños, chopped

Directions:

1. Set a suitable sized cooking pot over moderate heat and add the oil to heat.

2. Toss in the pork pieces and sauté for 4 minutes.

3. Stir in the garlic and onion, then stir-fry for 4 minutes until the onion is soft.

4. Add the remaining ingredients, then cover the pork soup.

5. Cook for 45 minutes until the pork is tender.

6. Serve warm.

Nutrition:

Calories 128

Total Fat 6.7 g

Saturated Fat 1 g

Cholesterol 0 mg

Sodium 883 mg

Carbohydrate 11.7 g

Dietary Fiber 2.3 g

Sugars 3.6 g

Protein 5.3 g

Calcium 35 mgPhosphorous 83 mgPotassium 286 mg

Crab Corn Chowder

Preparation Time: 5 Minutes

Cooking Time: 12 Minutes

Servings: 6

Ingredients:

- Six bacon slices
- Two celery ribs, diced
- One green bell pepper, diced
- One onion, diced
- One jalapeño pepper, seeded and diced
- 1 (32-oz.) container chicken broth
- Three tablespoons flour
- 3 cups corn kernels
- 1 lb. crabmeat, drained
- 1 cup whipping cream
- 1/4 teaspoon pepper

Directions:

1. Add the bacon to a wok and sear it until golden brown, then transfer to a plate.

2. Stir in the onion, celery, and bell pepper, then sauté until soft.

3. Add the corn, broth, crabmeat, cream, black pepper, and flour.

4. Mix well and cook, stirring slowly for 10 minutes.

5. Serve warm.

Nutrition:

Calories 330

Total Fat 15.5 g

Saturated Fat 6.8 g

Cholesterol 58 mg

Sodium 105 mg

Carbohydrate 33.5 g

Dietary Fiber 3.6 g

Sugars 9.3 g

Protein 16.7 g

Calcium 38 mg

Phosphorous 146 mg

Potassium 512 mg

Chicken Green Beans Soup

Preparation Time: 5 Minutes

Cooking Time: 25 Minutes

Servings: 4

Ingredients:

- 1 lb. chicken breasts, boneless, skinless, cubed
- 1 1/2 cups onion, sliced
- 1 1/2 cups celery, chopped
- One tablespoon olive oil
- 1 cup carrots, chopped
- 1 cup green beans, chopped
- Three tablespoons flour
- One teaspoon dried oregano
- Two teaspoons dried basil
- 1/4 teaspoon nutmeg
- One teaspoon thyme
- 32 oz. chicken broth
- 1/2 cup milk
- 2 cups frozen green peas

- 1/4 teaspoon black pepper

Directions:

1. Add the chicken to a skillet and sauté for 6 minutes, then remove it from the heat.

2. Warm up the olive oil in a pan and stir-fry the onion for 5 minutes.

3. Stir in the carrots, flour, green beans, basil, the sautéed chicken, thyme, oregano, and nutmeg.

4. Sauté for approximately 3 minutes, then transfer the ingredients to a large pan.

5. Add the milk and broth and cook until it boils.

6. Stir in the green peas and cook for 5 minutes.

7. Adjust seasoning with pepper and serve warm.

Nutrition:

Calories 277

Total Fat 9.6 g

Saturated Fat 2.4 g

Cholesterol 69 mg

Sodium 586 mg

Carbohydrate 17.3 g

Dietary Fiber 4.5 g

Sugars 6.4 g

Protein 29.5 g

Calcium 86 mg

Phosphorous 284 mg

Potassium 624 mg

Cream of Corn Soup

Preparation Time: 5 Minutes

Cooking Time: 10 Minutes

Servings: 3

Ingredients:

- Two tablespoons butter

- Two tablespoons flour

- 1/8 teaspoon black pepper

- 1 cup of water

- 1 cup liquid non-dairy creamer

- Two jars (4.5 oz. non-dairy creamer) strained baby corn

Directions:

1. Thaw the butter in a saucepan, then add the black pepper and flour.

2. Stir well until smooth, then add the water and creamer.

3. Mix well and cook until the soup bubbles.

4. Add the baby corn and mix well.

5. Serve.

Nutrition:

Calories 128

Total Fat 9.1 g

Saturated Fat 1.3 g

Cholesterol 0 mg

Sodium 185 mg

Carbohydrate 8.1 g

Dietary Fiber 0.2 g

Sugars 4 g

Protein 0.6 g

Calcium 6 mg

Phosphorous 293 mg

Potassium 11 mg

Cabbage Beef Borscht

Preparation Time: 5 Minutes

Cooking Time: 2 Hours

Servings: 12

Ingredients:

- Two tablespoons vegetable oil

- 3 lbs. beef short ribs

- 1/2 cup dry red wine

- 8 cups low-sodium chicken broth

- 1/2 tablespoon berries

- 1/2 tablespoon whole black peppercorns

- 1/2 tablespoon coriander seeds

- Two dill sprigs

- Two oregano sprigs

- Two parsley sprigs

- Two tablespoons unsalted butter

- Three beets (1 1/2 lbs.), peeled and diced

- One small rutabaga (1/2 lb.), peeled and diced

- One leek, diced

- One small onion, diced (1 cup)

- 1/2 lb. carrots, diced

- Two celery ribs, diced

- 1/2 head savoy cabbage (1 lb.), cored and shredded

- 7 oz. chopped tomatoes, canned

- 1/2 cup dry red wine

- Two tablespoons red wine vinegar

- Freshly ground pepper

- Sour cream

- Chopped dill

- Horseradish, grated, for serving

Directions:

1. Begin by placing the ribs in a large cooking pot and pour enough water to cover it.

2. Cover the beef pot and cook it on a simmer until it is tender, then shred it using a fork.

3. Add the olive oil, rutabaga, carrots, shredded cabbage, and the remaining ingredients to the cooking liquid in the pot.

4. Cover the cabbage soup and cook on low heat for 1 ½ hour.

5. Serve warm.

Nutrition:

Calories 537

Total Fat 45.5 g

Saturated Fat 19.8 g

Cholesterol 90 mg

Sodium 200 mg

Carbohydrate 10 g

Dietary Fiber 2.3 g

Sugars 5.1 g

Protein 18.7 g

Calcium 60 mg

Phosphorous 377 mg

Potassium 269 mg

Lemon Pepper Beef Soup

Preparation Time: 5 Minutes

Cooking Time: 35 Minutes

Servings: 6

Ingredients:

- 1 lb. lean ground beef
- 1/2 cup onion, chopped
- Two teaspoons lemon-pepper seasoning blend
- 1 cup beef broth
- 2 cups of water
- 1/3 cup white rice, uncooked
- 3 cups of frozen mixed vegetables
- One tablespoon sour cream
- Cooking oil

Directions:

1. Spray a saucepan with cooking oil and place it over moderate heat.

2. Toss in the onion and ground beef, and sauté until brown.

3. Stir in the broth, and the rest of the ingredients, then boil.

4. Reduce the heat to a simmer, then cover the soup to cook for

another 30 minutes.

5. Garnish with sour cream.

6. Enjoy.

Nutrition:

Calories 252

Total Fat 5.6 g

Saturated Fat 2.2 g

Cholesterol 68 mg

Sodium 213 mg

Carbohydrate 21.3 g

Dietary Fiber 4.3 g

Sugars 3.4 g

Protein 27.2 g

Calcium 42 mg

Phosphorous 359 mg

Potassium 211 mg

Vegetable
Recipes

Rutabaga Latkes

Preparation Time: 15 Minutes

Cooking Time: 7 Minutes

Servings: 4

Ingredients:

- One teaspoon hemp seed

- One teaspoon ground black pepper

- 7 oz rutabaga, grated

- ½ teaspoon ground paprika

- Two tablespoons coconut flour

- One egg, beaten

- One teaspoon olive oil

Directions:

1. Mix up together hemp seeds, ground black pepper, ground paprika, and coconut flour.

2. Then add grated rutabaga and beaten egg.

3. With the help of the fork, combine all the ingredients into the smooth mixture.

4. Preheat the skillet for 2-3 minutes over the high heat.

5. Then reduce the heat till medium and add olive oil.

6. With the help of the fork, place the small amount of rutabaga mixture in the skillet. Flatten it gently in the shape of latkes.

7. Cook the latkes for 3 minutes from each side.

8. After this, transfer them to the plate and repeat the same steps with the remaining rutabaga mixture.

Nutrition:

Calories 64

Fat 3.1

Fiber 3

Carbs 7.1

Protein 2.8

Glazed Snap Peas

Preparation Time: 10 Minutes

Cooking Time: 5 Minutes

Servings: 2

Ingredients:

- 1 cup snap peas

- Two teaspoon Erythritol

- One teaspoon butter, melted

- ¾ teaspoon ground nutmeg

- ¼ teaspoon salt

- 1 cup water for cooking

Directions:

1. Pour water into the pan. Add snap peas and bring them to boil.

2. Boil the snap peas for 5 minutes over medium heat.

3. Then drain water and chill the snap peas.

4. Meanwhile, whisk together ground nutmeg, melted butter, salt, and Erythritol.

5. Preheat the mixture in the microwave oven for 5 seconds.

6. Pour the sweet butter liquid over the snap peas and shake

them well.

7. The side dish should be served only warm.

Nutrition:

Calories 80

Fat 2.5

Fiber 3.9

Carbs 10.9

Protein 4

Steamed Collard Greens

Preparation Time: 10 Minutes

Cooking Time: 5 Minutes

Servings: 2

Ingredients:

- 2 cups Collard Greens
- One tablespoon lime juice
- One teaspoon olive oil
- One teaspoon sesame seed
- ½ teaspoon chili flakes
- 1 cup water for the steamer

Directions:

1. Chop collard greens roughly.

2. Pour water in the steamer and insert rack.

3. Place the steamer bowl, add collard greens, and close the lid.

4. Steam the greens for 5 minutes.

5. After this, transfer the steamed collard greens to the salad bowl.

6. Sprinkle it with the lime juice, olive oil, sesame seeds, and

chili flakes.

7. Mix up greens with the help of 2 forks and leave to rest for 10 minutes before serving.

Nutrition:

Calories 43

Fat 3.4

Fiber 1.7

Carbs 3.4

Protein 1.3

Baked Eggplant Slices

Preparation Time: 15 Minutes

Cooking Time: 15 Minutes

Servings: 3

Ingredients:

- One large eggplant, trimmed

- One tablespoon butter softened

- One teaspoon minced garlic

- One teaspoon salt

Directions:

1. Cut the eggplant and sprinkle it with salt. Mix up well and leave for 10 minutes to make the vegetable "give" bitter juice.

2. After this, dry the eggplant with a paper towel.

3. In the shallow bowl, mix up together minced garlic and softened butter.

4. Brush every eggplant slice with the garlic mixture.

5. Line the baking tray with baking paper—Preheat the oven to 355F.

6. Place the sliced eggplants in the tray to make one layer and

transfer it to the oven.

7. Bake the eggplants for 15 minutes. The cooked eggplants

will be tender but not soft!

Nutrition:

Calories 81

Fat 4.2

Fiber 6.5

Carbs 11.1

Protein 1.9

Pesto Avocado

Preparation Time: 10 Minutes

Cooking Time: 10 Minutes

Servings: 2

Ingredients:

- One avocado pitted, halved

- 1/3 cup Mozzarella balls, cherry size

- 1 cup fresh basil

- One tablespoon walnut

- ¼ teaspoon garlic, minced

- ¾ teaspoon salt

- ¾ teaspoon ground black pepper

- Four tablespoons olive oil

- 1 oz Parmesan, grated

- 1/3 cup cherry tomatoes

Directions:

1. Make pesto sauce: blend salt, minced garlic, walnuts, fresh basil, ground black pepper, and olive oil.

2. When the mixture is smooth, augment grated cheese and pulse it for 3 seconds more.

115

3. Then scoop ½ flesh from the avocado halves.

4. In the mixing bowl, mix up together mozzarella balls and

cherry tomatoes.

5. Add pesto sauce and shake it well.

6. Preheat the oven to 360F.

7. Fill the avocado halves with the cherry tomato mixture and

bake for 10 minutes.

Nutrition:

Calories 526

Fat 53.2

Fiber 7.8

Carbs 11.7

Protein 8.2

Vegetable Masala

Preparation Time: 10 Minutes

Cooking Time: 18 Minutes

Servings: 4

Ingredients:

- 2 cups green beans, chopped

- 1 cup white mushroom, chopped

- ¾ cup tomatoes, crushed

- One teaspoon minced garlic

- One teaspoon minced ginger

- One teaspoon chili flake

- One tablespoon garam masala

- One tablespoon olive oil

- One teaspoon salt

Directions:

1. Line the tray with parchment and preheat the oven to 360F.

2. Place the green beans and mushrooms in the tray.

3. Sprinkle the vegetables with crushed tomatoes, minced garlic and ginger, chili flakes, garam masala, olive oil, and salt.

4. Mix up well and transfer in the oven.

5. Cook vegetable masala for 18 minutes.

Nutrition:

Calories 60

Fat 30.7

Fiber 2.5

Carbs 6.4

Protein 2

Fast Cabbage Cakes

Preparation Time: 15 Minutes

Cooking Time: 10 Minutes

Servings: 2

Ingredients:

- 1 cup cauliflower, shredded

- One egg, beaten

- One teaspoon salt

- One teaspoon ground black pepper

- Two tablespoons almond flour

- One teaspoon olive oil

Directions:

1. Blend the shredded cabbage in the blender until you get cabbage rice.

2. Then, mix up cabbage rice with the egg, salt, ground black pepper, and almond flour.

3. Pour olive oil into the skillet and preheat it.

4. Then make the small cakes with the help of 2 spoons and place them in the hot oil.

5. Roast the cabbage cakes for 4 minutes from each side over

medium-low heat.

6. It is suggested to use a non-stick skillet.

Nutrition:

Calories 227

Fat 18.6

Fiber 4.5

Carbs 9.5

Protein 9.9

Cilantro Chili Burgers

Preparation Time: 10 Minutes

Cooking Time: 15 Minutes

Servings: 3

Ingredients:

- 1 cup red cabbage

- Three tablespoons almond flour

- One tablespoon cream cheese

- 1 oz scallions, chopped

- ½ teaspoon salt

- ½ teaspoon chili powder

- ½ cup fresh cilantro

Directions:

1. Chop red cabbage roughly and transfer in the blender.

2. Add fresh cilantro and blend the mixture until very smooth.

3. After this, transfer it to the bowl.

4. Add cream cheese, scallions, salt, chili powder, and almond flour.

5. Stir the mixture well.

6. Make three big burgers from the cabbage mixture or six small

burgers.

7. Line the baking tray with baking paper.

8. Place the burgers in the tray.

9. Bake the cilantro burgers for 15 minutes at 360F.

10. Flip the burgers onto another side after 8 minutes of cooking.

Nutrition:

Calories 182

Fat 15.3

Fiber 4.1

Carbs 8.5

Protein 6.8

Jicama Noodles

Preparation Time: 15 Minutes

Cooking Time: 7 Minutes

Servings: 6

Ingredients:

- 1-pound jicama, peeled

- Two tablespoons butter

- One teaspoon chili flake

- One teaspoon salt

- ¾ cup of water

Directions:

1. Spiralize jicama with the help of a spiralizer and place in jicama spirals in the saucepan.

2. Add butter, chili flakes, and salt.

3. Then add water and preheat the ingredients until the butter is melted.

4. Mix it up well.

5. Close the lid and cook noodles for 4 minutes over medium heat.

6. Stir the jicama noodles well before transferring them to the

serving plates.

Nutrition:

Calories 63

Fat 3.9

Fiber 3.7

Carbs 6.7

Protein 0.6

Crack Slaw

Preparation Time: 15 Minutes

Cooking Time: 10 Minutes

Servings: 6

Ingredients:

1 cup cauliflower rice

One tablespoon sriracha

One teaspoon tahini paste

One teaspoon sesame seed

One tablespoon lemon juice

One teaspoon olive oil

One teaspoon butter

½ teaspoon salt

2 cups coleslaw

Directions:

1. Toss the butter in the skillet and melt it.

2. Add cauliflower rice and sprinkle it with sriracha and tahini paste.

3. Mix up the vegetables and cook them for 10 minutes over medium heat. Stir them from time to time.

4. When the cauliflower is cooked, transfer it to the big plate.

5. Add coleslaw and stir gently.

6. Then sprinkle the salad with sesame seeds, lemon juice, olive oil, and salt.

7. Mix up well.

Nutrition:

Calories 76

Fat 5.8

Fiber 0.6

Carbs 6

Protein 1.1

Dessert Recipes

Dessert Cocktail

Preparation Time: 0 Minutes

Cooking Time: 1 Minute

Servings: 4

Ingredients:

- 1 cup of cranberry juice

- 1 cup of fresh ripe strawberries, washed and hull removed

- 2 tbsp of lime juice

- ¼ cup of white sugar

- Eight ice cubes

Directions:

1. Combine all the ingredients in a blender until smooth and creamy.

2. Pour the liquid into tall chilled glasses and serve cold.

Nutrition: Calories: 92 kcal Carbohydrate: 23.5 g Protein: 0.5 g Sodium: 3.62 mg

Potassium: 103.78 phosphorus: 17.86 dietary Fiber: 0.84 fat: 0.17 g

Baked Egg Custard

Preparation Time: 5 Minutes

Cooking Time: 25 Minutes

Servings: 4

Ingredients:

- Two medium eggs, at room temperature
- ¼ cup of semi-skimmed milk
- 3 tbsp of white sugar
- ½ tsp of nutmeg
- 1 tsp of vanilla extract

Directions:

1. Preheat your oven at 375 F/180C

2. Blend all the fixings in a mixing bowl and beat with a hand mixer for a few seconds until creamy and uniform.

3. Pour the mixture into lightly greased muffin tins.

4. Bake for 25-30 minutes or until the knife you place inside comes out clean.

Nutrition:

Calories: 96.56 kcal

Carbohydrate: 10.5 g

Protein: 3.5 g

Sodium: 37.75 mg

Potassium: 58.19 mg

Phosphorus: 58.76 mg

Dietary Fiber: 0.06 g

Fat: 2.91 g

Gumdrop Cookies

Preparation Time: 5 Minutes

Cooking Time: 12 Minutes

Servings: 25

Ingredients:

- ½ cup of spreadable unsalted butter

- One medium egg

- 1 cup of brown sugar

- 1 2/3 cups of all-purpose flour, sifted

- ¼ cup of milk

- 1 tsp vanilla

- 1 tsp of baking powder

- 15 large gumdrops, chopped finely

Directions:

1. Preheat the oven at 400F/195C.

2. Combine the sugar, butter, and egg until creamy.

3. Add the milk and vanilla and stir well.

4. Combine the flour with the baking powder in a different bowl.

Incorporate the sugar, butter mixture, and stir.

5. Add the gumdrops and place the mixture in the fridge for half

an hour.

6. Drop the dough with tablespoonful into a lightly greased baking or cookie sheet.

7. Bake for 10-12 minutes or until golden brown.

Nutrition:

Calories: 102.17 kcal

Carbohydrate: 16.5 g

Protein: 0.86 g

Sodium: 23.42 mg

Potassium: 45 mg

Phosphorus: 32.15 mg

Dietary Fiber: 0.13 g

Fat: 4 g

Pound Cake with Pineapple

Preparation Time: 5 Minutes

Cooking Time: 50 Minutes

Servings: 24

Ingredients:

- 3 cups of all-purpose flour, sifted

- 3 cups of sugar

- 1 ½ cups of butter

- Six whole eggs and three egg whites

- 1 tsp of vanilla extract

- 1 10. oz can of pineapple chunks, rinsed and crushed (keep the

- juice aside).

For the glaze:

- 1 cup of sugar

- One stick of unsalted butter or margarine

- Reserved juice from the pineapple

Directions:

1. Preheat the oven at 350F/180C.

2. Beat the sugar and the butter with a hand mixer until creamy

and smooth.

3. Slowly add the eggs (one or two every time) and stir well after pouring each egg.

4. Add the vanilla extract, follow up with the flour and stir well.

5. Add the drained and chopped pineapple.

6. Pour the mixture into a greased cake tin and bake for 45-50 minutes.

7. In a small saucepan, combine the sugar with the butter and pineapple juice. Stir every few seconds and bring to boil. Cook until you get creamy to a thick glaze consistency.

8. Pour the glaze over the cake, whereas still hot.

9. Let cook for at least 10 seconds and serve.

Nutrition:

Calories: 407.4 kcal

Carbohydrate: 79 g

Protein: 4.25 g

Sodium: 118.97 mg

Potassium: 180.32 mg

Phosphorus: 66.37 mg

Dietary Fiber: 2.25 gFat: 16.48 g

Apple Crunch Pie

Preparation Time: 5 Minutes

Cooking Time: 35 Minutes

Servings: 8

Ingredients:

Four large tart apples, peeled, seeded, and sliced

- ½ cup of all-purpose white flour

- 1/3 cup margarine

- 1 cup of sugar

- ¾ cup of rolled oat flakes

- ½ tsp of ground nutmeg

Directions:

1. Preheat the oven to 375F/180C.

2. Place the apples over a lightly greased square pan (around 7 inches).

3. Mix the rest of the fixings in a medium bowl and spread the batter over the apples.

4. Bake for 30-35 minutes or until the top crust has gotten golden brown.

5. Serve hot.

Nutrition:

Calories: 261.9 kcal

Carbohydrate: 47.2 g

Protein: 1.5 g

Sodium: 81 mg

Potassium: 123.74 mg

Phosphorus: 35.27 mg

Dietary Fiber: 2.81 g

Fat: 7.99 g

Easy Chocolate Pie Shell

Preparation Time: 5 Minutes

Cooking Time: 25 Minutes

Servings: 6

Ingredients:

- 3 cups of cocoa rice Krispies, crushed

- ½ stick of unsalted butter, melted

Directions:

1. Place crushed cocoa Krispies in a bowl with the melted butter.

Mix well with a spatula.

2. Spray an 8-9-inch pie pan with some low-calorie cooking spray

3. Press the mixture into the pan and even out with a spatula.

4. Let sit and chill for at least 30 minutes in the fridge before filling

it with chocolate or vanilla pudding.

Nutrition:

Calories: 113.1 kcal

Carbohydrate: 11.6 g

Protein: 0.88 g Sodium: 122.98 mg

Potassium: 17.3 phosphorus: 18.23 dietary Fiber: 0.04 fat: 7.82 g

Strawberry and Mint Sorbet

Preparation Time: 0 Minutes

Cooking Time: 1 Minute

Servings: 3-4

- Ingredients:

- ¼ cup of white sugar

- 1 cup of frozen or fresh, cut strawberries

- 1 tbsp of lime juice

- ¼ cup of water

- One ¼ cup of crushed ice

- A few mint leaves

Directions:

1. Pulse and crush the ice in a heavy-duty blender.

2. Add the remaining ingredients and raise the speed to crush

until no lumps of ice are left.

3. Optionally add a few mint leaves for garnishing.

Nutrition:

Calories: 93.34 kcal

Carbohydrate: 32 g

Protein: 0.33 g

Sodium: 2.12 mg

Potassium: 113.02 mg

Phosphorus: 10.24 mg

Dietary Fiber: 1.56 g

Fat: 0.067 g

Easy Chocolate Fudge

Preparation Time: 5 Minutes

Cooking Time: 10 Minutes

Servings: 12

Ingredients:

- 2/3 cup of half and half cream

- 1 cup of white granulated sugar

- 1 cups of semi-sweet chocolate chip cookies

- 1 cup of mini marshmallows

- 1 tsp of vanilla extract

Directions:

1. Grease with cooking spray a square pie pan (around 9 inches).

2. Mix the half-and-half cream with the sugar in a medium saucepan. Bring to a boil and adjust to medium heat.

3. Take off the heat and add the chocolate chips, the marshmallows, and the vanilla extract. Stir well with a spatula until everything is melted.

4. Quickly transfer the mixture into the pie pan. Let cool for at least 10 minutes and cut into square pieces, around 3x2" each. It will make 18-20 pieces.

Nutrition:

Calories: 52.4 kcal

Carbohydrate: 17.58 g

Protein: 3.18 g

Sodium: 153.47 mg

Potassium: 100.52 mg

Phosphorus: 38.63 mg

Dietary Fiber: 1.35 g

Fat: 21.3 g

Lemon Mousse

Preparation Time: 10 Minutes Plus Chill Time

Cooking Time: 10 Minutes

Servings: 4

Ingredients:

- 1 cup coconut cream

- 8 ounces cream cheese, soft

- ¼ cup fresh lemon juice

- Three pinches salt

- One teaspoon lemon liquid stevia

Directions:

1. Preheat your oven to 350 °F

2. Grease a ramekin with butter

3. Beat cream, cream cheese, fresh lemon juice, salt, and lemon liquid stevia in a mixer

4. Pour batter into ramekin

5. Bake for 10 minutes, then transfer the mousse to a serving glass

6. Let it chill for 2 hours and serve

7. Enjoy!

142

Nutrition:

Calories: 395

Fat: 31 g

Carbohydrates: 3 g

Protein: 5 g

Jalapeno Crisp

Preparation Time: 10 Minutes

Cooking Time: 1 Hour and 15 Minutes

Servings: 20

Ingredients:

- 1 cup sesame seeds

- 1 cup sunflower seeds

- 1 cup flaxseeds

- ½ cup hulled hemp seeds

- Three tablespoons Psyllium husk

- One teaspoon salt

- One teaspoon baking powder

- 2 cups of water

Directions:

1. Preheat your oven to 350 °F

2. Take your blender and add seeds, baking powder, salt, and

Psyllium husk

3. Blend well until a sand-like texture appears

4. Stir in water and mix until a batter form

5. Allow the batter to rest for 10 minutes until a dough-like thick

mixture forms

6. Pour the dough onto a cookie sheet lined with parchment paper

7. Spread it evenly, making sure that it has a thickness of ¼ inch thick all around

8. Bake for 75 minutes in your oven

9. Remove and cut into 20 spices

10. Let them cool for 30 minutes and enjoy it!

Nutrition:

Calories: 156

Fat: 13 g

Carbohydrates: 2 g

Protein: 5 g

Raspberry Popsicle

Preparation Time: 2 Hours

Cooking Time: 15 Minutes

Servings: 4

Ingredients:

- 1 ½ cups raspberries

- 2 cups of water

Directions:

1. Take a pan and fill it up with water

2. Add raspberries

3. Place it over medium heat and bring to water to a boil

4. Lessen the temperature and simmer for 15 minutes

5. Remove heat and pour the mix into Popsicle molds

6. Add a popsicle stick and let it chill for 2 hours

7. Serve and enjoy!

Nutrition:

Calories: 58

Fat: 0.4 g

Carbohydrates: 0 g

Protein: 1.4 g